Dr. Sebi Nutritional Guide for Erectile Dysfunction

How to confidently regain Strong & Healthy Erection via Alkaline and Detox Diet & Herbs.

FRED WRIGHT

This book is not written to promote sexual immoralities, but written to help enlightened men on how they can treat Erectile Dysfunction.

TABLE OF CONTENTS

DR. SEBI NUTRITIONAL GUIDE FOR ERECTILE DYSFUNCTION I

INTRODUCTION 6

CHAPTER ONE..11

THE MANHOOD 11

THINGS I NEED TO KNOW ABOUT MY MANHOOD?....................................12

MAJOR FUNCTIONS OF THE MANHOOD. 13

CHAPTER TWO...18

STRUCTURE OF PENILE SYSTEM...18

COMPOSITION OF PENILE SYSTEM? 20

BEFORE ERECTION? 23

CHAPTER THREE 26

ERECTILE DYSFUNCTION – IMPOTENCE 26

PROCESSES INVOLVE BEFORE ERECTION 27

THE GLOBAL RISE OF ERECTILE DYSFUNCTION 28

OTHER SEXUAL RELATED PROBLEMS 30

LIKELY SYMPTOMS OF ERECTILE DYSFUNCTION 30

LIKELY CAUSES OF ERECTILE DYSFUNCTION? 32

Tips to prevent erectile dysfunction. 38

COMMON SUPPLEMENTS AND DRUGS FOR THE TREATMENT OF ERECTILE DYSFUNCTION 42

CHAPTER FOUR..44

FOODS TO BUILD HEALTHY PENILE SYSTEMS..44

ALKALINE DIET..44

SPINACH 46

ALMONDS...47

YOGURT 48

TOMATOES... 49

POTATOES 50

SARDINES 50

BLUEBERRIES.. 51

AVOCADOS... 52

WHOLE GRAINS.. 53

A GLASS OF RED WINE 54

WATERMELON 54

CHAPTER FOUR...**56**

How To Build Blood for Good Erection 56

CHAPTER FIVE **62**

DOES VIAGRA HELPS?.. 62

The use of Viagra 64

The compositional Ingredients of Viagra? 65

How long does it take to start the effect? 66

How long does Viagra take to maintain effect? 66

Factors that may affect the lasting effect of Viagra and some other ED

drugs 67

Precaution on the right dose of Viagra 71

Precautions on when Not to Take Viagra or any other ED Drugs 72

Health conditions that may prevent you from using Viagra. 75

Drugs that Interact with Viagra? 76

What to do when you take an overdose? 76

Is Viagra safe for health?... 77

What Are the Possible Side Effects of Viagra? 77

The most common side effect of Viagra 79

The common side effect of Viagra 79

Uncommon side effect 81

Rare side effects.. 82

ABOUT THE AUTHOR **85**

ACKNOWLEDGEMENTS 86

INTRODUCTION

Dr. Sebi was a great knowledge and experienced herbalist, who sufficiently and thoroughly gather herbs and therapeutic alkaline diet that can help maintain good health system. In course of his life, he had experienced erectile dysfunction which is the most pronounced men sexual problem. This ailment set him on a path to naturally treat this sickness by using vast knowledge in herb mixture, in order to regain is sexual fitness and, more so help others treat the ailment.

As it is known that the drive to engage in sexual activities has grown so much that young men and women cannot but satisfy their desire when they need it. But over time, the reach for libido has been challenging for some men because of this general sexual problem - erectile dysfunction. Erectile dysfunction is a sickness that is rampant among men as they aged. In some men, it may be as a result of stress and, in others – factors beyond their reach that will be extensively discussed in the later chapter. Dr. Sebi understands that, many go as far as taken stimulant, which will only work during the time of the intercourse and it becomes inactive after sexual activity. As time goes on, he noticed that some of these drugs either affect the other body system or render man inactive without their use. Erectile dysfunction has kept men and women on long research to get an aid that can help improve their sex life. With careful and thorough search, Dr. Sebi gathered a group of curative herbs and alkaline diets for erectile dysfunction.

Deep thought for a man going through erectile dysfunction …

To lose or not attain erection during sexual intercourse can cause a lot of misdemeanors between the two sexual parties such as break relationship, frustration, misunderstanding, adultery, and fornication and sometimes divorce. It will be challenging to try to convince any woman about why you lose your erection during sexual intercourse. Most of the time, it left them in an uncontrollable state since some of them might be closer or in orgasm.

Erectile dysfunction (ED) is the inability to reach and maintain penile erection sufficient for satisfactory sexual activity. Over the years Erectile Dysfunction has had a lot of pronouncing irregularities in men to such an extent of resulting into loss of self-esteem, broken relationship, divorce, lack of self – confidence tension, and more.

When a man self- esteem is low, he develops a high tendency of anxiety, stress, loneliness and depression resulting into problems with friends and even his partner.

and all these will not support the recovery processes from the condition.

The pronouncement of Erectile Dysfunction is recorded to be associated with age increase. Complete ED has an estimated prevalence of about 5% in men who are of 40 years of age and 15% at age 70 years.

The broad insights into the mechanism of penile erection have led to the development of several methods of treating problems associated with penile erections, which may include erectile dysfunction. However, this book shall be discussing all penile system which may includes

- *Its structures.*

- *The problems of penile erection.*

- *How penile problems can be prevented.*

- *How penile problems can be treated.*

- *Genuine ways of treating penile problems.*

- *Foods you can eat that help maintain a healthy penile system or sex life.*

- *What should you abstain from to prevent penile erection problems?*

- *Things you do but don't know gradually affect your sex life.*

Dr. Sebi's experiences during the days he suffers from erectile dysfunction and how he treated it naturally will save you a lot of heartaches from your wife. Build a right home for yourself by getting this series.

Chapter One

THE MANHOOD

One of the reasons for existence is to **_Reproduce_**. As we were birthed, so we are meant to reproduce. However, if you have decided to be a eunuch, that does not dispute the facts that you are a man that have qualities and organs that can make you reproduce. Have you ever thought about this fact, **_"if the manhood of your father was inactive or impotent, will you be birthed to live on this planet earth?_**

As a lot of people may shy away from this topic, most especially in the religious sect, probably with the thought of it being private discussion. Many folks keep dying on the run to finding sustainable solution. Some homes are broken, quite a number of husbands and wives are divorced, and relationship are experiencing hell while on earth because of the ignorance of their mind. They think it is a sacred topic which must not be discussed in a general assembly. Religious sects broadened the myth "it *is a private and sacred topic*" and their followers keep swimming in the pool of unsuccessful marriage or relationships.

Do I mean it should be addressed unguided, or anyhow without taking caution? NO. This is what I'm saying, do not die in the ignorance of the secrecy of sexual problems, but understand all you need to know about how you can build muscular strength for good sex life. It will save you a lot of worries.

Things I need to know about My Manhood?

If you are a man, check-in between the upper end (head) of your two thigh bones (femurs) or between the top ends of your legs at the hip region you will observe a tube-like structure pointing heads down. Generally, it is known to be (Penis).

The *manhood* is a male erectile organ of copulation, sometimes called the Private male part that helps in the discharge of urine (the liquid waste product of the body) and Semen (also known as sperm, whitish liquid) ejaculate during sexual activity. From the statement above, it can be deduced that manhood serves two primary functions in man – as waste disposal and as a life-giver.

Major functions of the Manhood.

- **A source of Reproduction:** The first step for a man to achieve this function is the ability of his manhood to erect. Erection is significant when it comes to the secretion of semen containing sperm cells for the fertilization of ovules. Without the production of semen or sperm cells in the semen – azoospermia and the insemination of sperms with the ovules, there will not be recreation. If a man is not impotent – the inability to get and maintain an erection, you will be able to satisfy your wife sexually, thereby building a happy home for yourself and stress-free environs in your family. Aside from recreation or fruitfulness, there is a satisfying pleasure you get from ejaculation or orgasm during sexual activities. When a man is healthy, the manhood gives him a satisfying moment with his wife. From when he is sexually aroused or stimulated, to gaining a penile erection, to penetration, orgasm, and ejaculation.

• **Waste disposal channel:** In the structure of the body, there are different channels at which waste are being passed out, which may include:

- Skin pores; sweat

- Nose; mucus

- Anus; faeces

- Sometimes mouth; phlegm

- Penis; urine.

Urination is the discharge of urine from the urinary bladder through the urethra out of the body system. It is a form of excretion. It's also recognized medically as voiding, micturition uresis, or, not often, emiction, and acknowledged colloquially by using various names which includes weeing, peeing, pissing (this name most times are commonly used by children).

In wholesome people, the manner of urination is termed to be a voluntary action. In toddlers, some aged individuals, and people with a neurological ailment, urination can also occur as a reflex action. It is usual for grown-up persons to urinate as much as seven times in the day. That doesn't mean you have a disease. But it is highly desirable to take caution on your body system, because urethra disease may affect the maximum performance of your sex life. Later chapters will discuss those urethra diseases, preventions, and cure.

A man should be aware that women generally take longer to reach orgasm than men. Averagely it takes women ten to twenty minutes during sexual activity while men only take two to three minutes. Most women need more than just penetration, and they also need clitoral stimulation. So how does this work? The clitoris enlarges and moves its position, the pelvic area swells with blood and genital muscles tighten. Orgasm reverses this process by releasing that built-up tension and causes muscle contractions in the vagina, pelvic floor, anus, and uterus. Women typically have six to ten contractions per orgasms compare to four to six for men. At orgasm, you feel happy, and this is the pleasure men and women derived in sex in addition to reproduction. At this stage, your brain releases endorphins and oxytocin. Then for maximum sexual pleasure, a man

penis should be in a proper state.

Chapter Two

STRUCTURE OF PENILE SYSTEM

The penile system is structured in such a way that it consists of the penis, testes, scrotum, epididymis, vas deferens, prostate and seminal vesticles. This is further summarised into Urinary and the reproductive system. The penis and the urethra function in the urinary system and their role cannot be sideline when reproductive system come to play. Additionally, the reproductive system is made up of the testicles, scrotum, prostate, seminal vesicles and vas deferens.

The penis is structured in a way that it has three cylindrical shaped tissue, and these tissues are affected during erection. We have two large Corpora cavernosa lying side by side and the Corpus spongiosum which surrounds the urethra. When these tissues are filled with blood, erection takes place.

Anatomy of the Penis

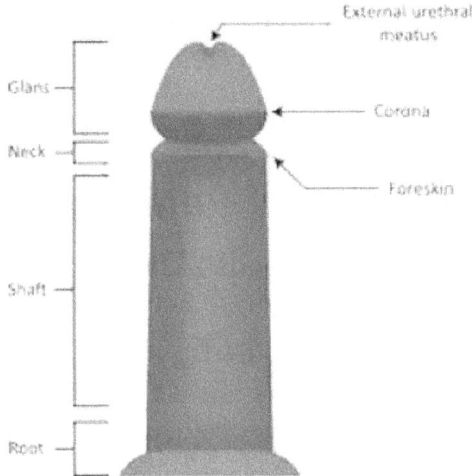

External urethral meatus

Glans

Corona

Neck

Foreskin

Shaft

Root

Comprehensive Penile System

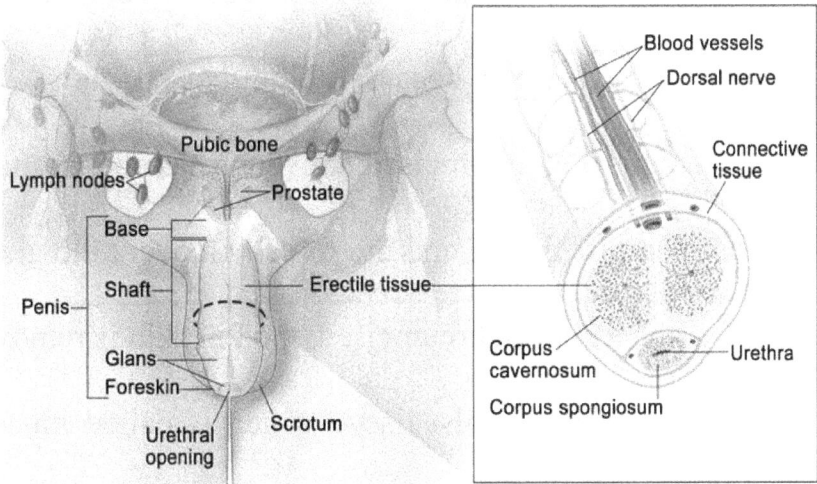

Pubic bone

Lymph nodes

Prostate

Base

Shaft

Penis

Erectile tissue

Glans

Foreskin

Urethral opening

Scrotum

Blood vessels

Dorsal nerve

Connective tissue

Corpus cavernosum

Corpus spongiosum

Urethra

From the figures above, you can understand the structure of

the penile system. The penis serves as a male sex organ that reaches its full size during the puberty stage. Additionally, it acts as a tube for urine (being a waste product) to leave the body system.

Composition of Penile system?

- *Glans:* The glans is also known as the head of the penis. You can check back the figures to see how the glans look. In the middle of the glans, there is an opening of the urethra (this is the tube where urine and semen are passed out of the body). The name "glans penis" was coined from a Latin word "**Acorn**" because of the shape of the glans. When a man is uncircumcised, the glans has a pink cover, mucosa – moist tissue, and the foreskin covers the glans. While when a man is circumcised, the foreskin is removed surgically, and the moist tissue which is called mucosa changes into dry skin.

- *Corpus Spongiosum:* This is a column of tissue that runs along the front of the penis and ends at the glans.

It is sponge-like in shape. It is located below the two-column of tissues of corpus cavernosum. The urethra runs through it, and it opens when it fills with blood during an erection. It is a smaller region when compared to the two-column of tissues of corpus cavernosum.

- **Corpus cavernosum:** These are two columns of tissues located at the sides of the penis. They perform the duty of allowing the flow of blood during an erection. These tissues have in their middle cavernosal arteries, which are filled with blood to cause an erection in the penis. There is a muscle that surrounds the corpus cavernosum that enables the penis to erect and contract during the ejaculation of semen.

- **Urethra:** Corpus Spongiosum is a column of tissue that has in it the urethra – which allows the passage of urine from the body system. This duct – urethra, allows the transportation of urine from the bladder out of the body during urination. There is a muscular structure called urethra sphincter, and it helps hold the urine in the bladder until it is ready for release.

Since the urethra is part of the reproductive system, its structure in the male reproductive system is different from that of the female. The male urethra can be divided into three (3) sections, and they are;

o   The topmost part within the prostate called the prostatic urethra.

o   The part within the urethra sphincter called the membranous urethra.

o   The lowest and the longest part of the penis called the spongy urethra. The spongy urethra, which is the lowest and the most extended section additionally has some other subdivisions, which include the following;

the periprostatic urethra, which is located at the neck of the bladder, the fossa navicularis, pendulous urethra, and bulbous urethra.

The three divisions above are categorized into anterior and posterior regions. The anterior part is made up of the *spongy urethra*, while the posterior part is made up of *prostatic urethra and the membranous urethra.*

The male urethra is about 8 inches (20cm) long, and this runs through the length of the penis, and it runs through the centre of the prostate (prostate gland), from the bladder to the penis, and the seminal ducts run from the testes, and it is connected to the urethra at each side. These functions make the urethra a part for the passage of both the urine and semen.

Before Erection?

Before erection occurs, the nerves in the penis receive an impulse from the brain and cause the relaxation of the muscles around the corpus cavernosum. The relaxation of these muscles creates an opening space for blood to flow into the corpus cavernosum. The pressure of the blood makes the penis expand and restrict the veins from returning the blood. Once the blood in the corpus cavernosum is entombed, the muscles in the tissue help to sustain an erection — the penis contract when the muscles in the penis disallow the flow of blood into the corpora cavernosa.

The female urethra

When you compare male urethra with the female urethra, they have some differences in structure. The female urethra is shorter in length than the male – it is 1.5 inches long (4cm). It starts its length from the neck of the bladder and opens outside after running through the urethral spinster. This makes the path urine passes in female to be more direct than that of male, which is curved. The urethra

in a female is enclosed within the vaginal walls, and it

opens between the labia.

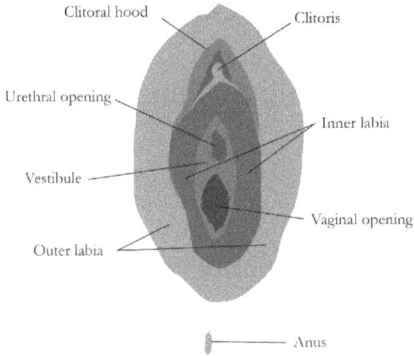

Chapter Three

ERECTILE DYSFUNCTION – IMPOTENCE

Erectile dysfunction is the inability to sustain a strong erection require to have satisfying sexual intercourse between a male and a female. Erectile dysfunction is also known as impotence.

Sometimes ED is related to stress problems with the sexual partner or transient psychological factors. A lot of men experience ED after times of stress. Constant occurrence of ED can be a sign of health issues that need to be attended to or requires treatment. It can also be a result of emotional instability or relationship difficulties that requires the attention of the right counselling to overcome. Some current therapeutic approach given to a patient who has erectile dysfunction includes the vacuum constriction device, penile prosthesis implantation or intracavernosal injections with vasodilating agents. include They are far from satisfactory for most patients, and some of these have limitations to their use

It must be understood that ejaculatory capacity, desire, and orgasmic capacity may not be affected even while suffering from erectile dysfunction or may be deficient to some extent and add to the sense of low performance during sexual activity. Erectile dysfunction can vary in man, and may range from a partial decrease in penile rigidity to full erectile failure. ED may also occur a few times in a specific period or cannot be able to gain an erection at all.

Processes Involve Before Erection

Attaining an erection is an intricate process that involves the sending of messages through nerves to the blood vessels present in the penis to allow the increase in the flow of blood.

The Messages sent to the spinal cord from nerves leave the lower spinal cord and cause the blood vessels that enter the spongy tissue - corpus cavernosum of the penis to dilate and allows the inflow of blood. There are two tubes of spongy tissue that run along the length of the penis. A tough fibrous, partly elastic outer cover surrounds this spongy material. When stimulated by the message sent through nerves, the spongy tissue aligns itself so that more blood will flow into the penis. The veins that run through the outer shield of the penis then compresses and resist the blood from flowing out of the penis. As the blood is hindered from leaving, the penis is filled with blood and stretches within the outer coverage, giving rise to an erection.

The Global Rise of Erectile Dysfunction

Erectile dysfunction is rampant among men, and its growth is increasing in this age as men grow older. During research by an Australian sometimes ago, his survey revealed that out of five (5) men over 40 years of age, a minimum of one has erectile dysfunction problem and out of ten (10), it was discovered that a minimum of 5 could not attain an erection at all. With this study, it was also realized that as ages increase, the chances of geometry growth of erectile dysfunction in men is high. Then you can also judge by the number of those buying erectile dysfunction's drugs – such as Viagra, Cialis, Levitra, and so on. From statistics of the Viagra sold annually, the daily number of sales of Viagra is higher when you compare to other erectile dysfunction drugs, and the annual sale aside from those buying other manufacturer products is hugely growing. This can equally bring us to the conclusion that the number of those that have this problem is much, and they increase daily.

Other Sexual Related Problems

It is highly pertinent not to be confused about erectile dysfunction and other sexual problems. Some men have little interest in sex (low libido) but have normal erections. And also, some men can get an erection but find it hard to ejaculate or get to reach an orgasm. Some have premature ejaculation – where they ejaculate early during sex or retrograde (dry) ejaculation – where semen flows back into the bladder rather than out of the penis during ejaculation. Each of these problems needs a different approach to diagnosis and treatment.

In a nutshell, a man must understand his major sexual problem because of not all male sexual issues resulting from erectile dysfunction. You need to know about your problem before you are treated, or purchase erectile dysfunction drug like Viagra.

Likely Symptoms of Erectile Dysfunction

Before concluding on friend advice on the supplement to take to energize your sex life, decide out of frustration or perceive without required knowledge, you need to know those symptoms that go alongside with the growth or effect of Erectile Dysfunction. These may include the following,

- Difficulty achieving an erection: One of the primary symptoms of ED is the inability to get an erection firm enough during sexual activity with your partner. This may involve struggling to achieve an erection or having an erection that is not firm or sustained

- Struggling to get an erection during sexual play: Has it gotten to the extent of sweating without erection during sexual activity with your partner? Once you start noticing this, take the necessary steps.

- You cannot maintain an erection during sexual intercourse.

- Little interest in sex.

If you begin to notice any of these symptoms, then you have to see your doctor for you to know the actual problem.

- Premature or delayed ejaculation: While not directly related to achieving or maintaining an erection, erectile dysfunction can sometimes be associated with problems in ejaculation. This can manifest as premature ejaculation (ejaculating too soon) or delayed ejaculation (difficulty ejaculating).

If you begin to notice any of these symptoms, then you have to see your doctor for you to know the actual problem.

Likely Causes of Erectile Dysfunction?

There are several causes of erectile dysfunction. These causes could be a result of physical, mental or emotional instabilities. There are a lot of factors that can affect a man's ability to get and maintain a penile erection. It may be a combination of physical and psychological factors, which may result in two or more elements, a sign of another serious, but in some cases, undiagnosed health issues, or sometimes there may not be an apparent reason as to what causes it. Some causes are listed below.

Intrusion with the function of nerve: *when you begin to notice some health problem affecting your nerve, then shift your thought to your erection. Some of these problems are;*

- Alzheimer's disease

- Diabetic neuropathy

- Developing a lot of scleroses

- Spinal cord problems

- Undergone a Pelvic surgery – prostate, bowel

- Parkinson's disease

Reduction in the flow of blood;

- Atherosclerosis – narrows arteries.

Excessive or unguided use of drugs, alcohol, and medicines.

- Alcohol and drug abuse

- Medicines used to treat: – Hypertension (high blood pressure), Psychiatric disorders, Prostate cancer.

Psychosocial factors such as listed below;

- Stress and anxiety: High levels of stress and anxiety can interfere with sexual arousal and performance.

- Depression: Feelings of sadness, hopelessness, and low self-esteem associated with depression can contribute to ED.

- Relationship issues: Problems within a relationship, communication difficulties, or unresolved conflicts can impact sexual function.

- Performance anxiety: Fear of not being able to perform sexually or satisfy a partner can lead to erectile difficulties.

- Anxiety

- Upbringing and sexual attitude

- Relationship problems

- Financial pressures.

- Unemployment issues

- Being Depressed

- Psychiatric imbalances

Metabolic problems interfering with blood vessel function (endothelial dysfunction)

- Diabetes

- Hypertension (high blood pressure)

- Obesity

- High cholesterol

- Cigarette smoking

- Sleep apnoea

Endocrine issues

- Thyroid disease

- Acromegaly – a condition caused by too much growth hormone

- sperm [spermatogenesis])

- Cortisone excess

- Hypogonadism – a condition where the testes are not able to make enough testosterone [androgen deficiency]

Urological issues

- Peyronie's disease

- Pelvic trauma

Lifestyle Factors

Unhealthy lifestyle choices can contribute to erectile dysfunction. These may include;

• Smoking: Smoking damages blood vessels and restricts blood flow, which can affect erectile function.

• Excessive alcohol consumption: Chronic alcohol abuse can lead to hormonal imbalances and nerve damage, contributing to ED.

• Substance abuse: The use of illicit drugs, such as cocaine or opioids, can affect sexual function.

• Sedentary lifestyle: Lack of physical activity and exercise can contribute to obesity, cardiovascular problems, and ED.

• Poor diet: A diet high in processed foods, saturated fats, and refined sugars can lead to obesity, diabetes, and other health conditions that can contribute to erectile dysfunction.

Tips to prevent erectile dysfunction.

Erectile dysfunction (ED) can have various causes, including physical, psychological, and lifestyle factors. While it's not always possible to prevent ED entirely, there are several steps you can take to reduce the risk or delay its onset. Here are some ways to prevent or minimize the occurrence of erectile dysfunction:

1. Maintain a healthy lifestyle: Adopting healthy habits can significantly lower the risk of developing ED. Focus on:

 - Regular exercise: Engage in physical activity, such as brisk walking, jogging, swimming, or cycling, for at least 30 minutes most days of the week. Exercise promotes blood circulation and overall cardiovascular health, which are essential for erectile function.

- Healthy diet: Consume a balanced diet rich in fruits, vegetables, whole grains, lean proteins, and healthy fats. Limit processed foods, sugary snacks, and excessive alcohol consumption. A healthy diet supports overall cardiovascular health and helps maintain a healthy weight.

- Maintain a healthy weight: Obesity is linked to an increased risk of ED. If you are overweight, losing weight through a combination of regular exercise and a healthy diet can improve erectile function.

2. Manage chronic conditions: Certain chronic conditions, such as diabetes, high blood pressure, and heart disease, can contribute to ED. Take the necessary steps to manage these conditions effectively, including:

- Regular medical check-ups and screenings

- Consistent medication adherence

- Following a recommended treatment plan

- Monitoring and controlling blood sugar levels and blood pressure.

3. Stop smoking: Smoking damages blood vessels and impairs blood flow, which can contribute to erectile dysfunction. If you smoke, consider quitting. Seek support from healthcare professionals or support groups to assist you in your efforts to quit smoking.

4. Limit alcohol consumption: Excessive alcohol intake can affect sexual function. Limit your alcohol consumption and try to avoid excessive or binge drinking.

5. Manage stress and psychological factors: Psychological factors like stress, anxiety, and depression can contribute to ED. Find healthy ways to manage stress, such as engaging in relaxation techniques (e.g., deep breathing, meditation, yoga), pursuing hobbies, spending time with loved ones, and seeking professional help if needed.

6. Communicate with your partner: Open and honest communication with your partner about sexual expectations, desires, and concerns can help reduce anxiety and improve intimacy.

7. Practice safe sex: Protecting yourself from sexually transmitted infections (STIs) can help prevent complications that might lead to erectile dysfunction. Use condoms consistently and correctly, especially with new or multiple sexual partners.

8. Get enough sleep: Poor sleep patterns and sleep disorders have been linked to erectile dysfunction. Aim for a sufficient amount of quality sleep each night to support overall health and sexual function.

9. Avoid illegal drugs: Illicit drug use, such as cocaine, marijuana, and opioids, can contribute to erectile dysfunction. Stay away from these substances to protect your sexual health.

10. Seek professional help: If you experience persistent or worsening erectile dysfunction, consult a healthcare professional. They can help identify any underlying causes and recommend appropriate treatments or therapies.

COMMON SUPPLEMENTS AND DRUGS FOR THE TREATMENT OF ERECTILE DYSFUNCTION

Since erectile dysfunction common among men. Some men have seen it as a general problem, and have custom their mind to some erectile dysfunction pills anytime they want to have a sex play with their wife. Drugs can help boost your energy, attain and maintain an erection, but it also has some adverse effect in your body as times go on. The most generally sold drug is Viagra, and some others will later be mention. But my emphasis will be dominant on this drug because of its extensive use, and as a case study because the erectile dysfunction drugs work almost similarly in function. Here are some examples of medications used for the treatment of erectile dysfunction; Cialis, Viagra, sildenafil, Staxyn, Tadalafil, Levitra, Caverject impulse, vardenafil, alprostadil, Edex, Stendra, Caverject, Muse, Avanafil. Examples of supplements that are men use to boost erection are; horny goat weed, yohimbine, damiana, and so on.

Chapter Four

FOODS TO BUILD HEALTHY PENILE SYSTEMS

Alkaline Diet

A good alkaline diet includes raw soups, vegetables, low carb or sugar, high-fat green, salads, oils and alkaline salts. Your alkaline diet plan can be on full time basis or periodic to build your penile system. when alkaline base food is consumed, the energy levels of the body system increases significantly, thus increases the response of the penis for erection. The combination of a standard alkaline diet would be 20% cooked food such as buckwheat, quinoa, millet or sometimes meat or fish and 80% alkaline oils and vegetables.

The following are some alkaline options for you.

Carbohydrate

- Soaked seeds/nuts.

- coconut or almond milk.

- Gluten-free porridge/cereal with hemp.

- sourdough spelt bread toasted with guacamole, salad avocado, almond butter.

- Millet, buckwheat, quinoa with salad, soup, vegetables, spices.

- Sweet potato, squash, pumpkin – prepare with vegetable curry and consume with salad. Yiu can as well have with steamed peas, broccoli, tomato, avocado e.t.c

Salads

Take salad with good oil, lemon, salt and small avocado.

Avocado and Juice

You can make a composition of a green vegetable juice mix with alkaline water and grind an avocado into the juice. Some green vegetable juice you can prepare include; cucumber, rocket, spinach, broccoli, watercress, cabbage. Then you mix avocado with the green vegetable juice.

Cinnamon smoothie

This is a mixture of avocado, one-fourth teaspoon of coconut oil, Alkaline water and one teaspoon of cinnamon – Ceylon cinnamon.

You can always take a raw chocolate, ripe fruit on empty stomach.

The following foods are also very important to build a good penile system.

SPINACH

Spinach is a super source of folate, a known blood flow-booster. Folic acid plays a critical role in male sexual function and a deficiency in folic acid has been linked Trusted Source to erectile dysfunction.

Cooked spinach contains 66 percent of your daily folic acid requirement per cup, making it one of the most folate-rich foods around. Additionally, spinach contains a fair amount of magnesium, which also helps improve and stimulate blood flow and has been shown as a trusted Source to boost testosterone levels.

Spinach is also good for penile health. It is a good source of folic acid which may help prevent erectile dysfunction. It also contains magnesium which has been shown to boost testosterone.

ALMONDS

Almonds contain zinc, selenium, and vitamin E, which are vitamins and minerals that seem to be important for sexual health and reproduction. Selenium can help with infertility issues and, with vitamin E, may help heart health. Zinc is a mineral that helps produce men's sex hormones and can boost libido.

Compared to all other nuts, almonds are the most packed with nutrients and beneficial components. Now all you need to do is to at about 8-10 almonds a day. You can either eat soaked almonds or crush it and add to your morning salad or garnish your dishes, it is beneficial in any way you use it.

YOGURT

Improved digestion. Yogurt contains probiotic bacteria, which are primarily known for their ability to promote digestive health.

According to the Harvard School of Public Health, several of the strains of probiotic bacteria found in yogurt may help prevent or treat digestive difficulties including indigestion, diarrhea, irritable bowel syndrome and Crohn's disease. Yogurt's probiotics can also promote regular bowel movements, better immune system functioning and improved vitamin, mineral and nutrient absorption.

According to Livestrong, if the results of studies conducted on male mice are any indication, yogurt may also have sexual benefits for men. Science suggests that certain dairy products, including yogurt, can help obese men lose weight. Finally, yogurt, and especially Greek yogurt, is a rich source of high-quality, muscle-building protein.

TOMATOES

Tomatoes have been linked to lowering men's risk of stroke, helping fight prostate cancer, and preserving brain power with age. Heating tomatoes significantly increases their levels of lycopene, the chemical that can up antioxidant levels.

Lycopene – a nutrient found in tomatoes – may boost sperm quality, a study has suggested. Healthy men who took the equivalent of two tablespoons of (concentrated) tomato puree a day as a supplement were found to have better quality sperm. Male infertility affects up to half of couples who cannot conceive.

POTATOES

Potatoes are an excellent source of potassium, a nutrient most people don't consume enough of, which can help regulate your blood pressure. They're a good source of vitamin C and vitamin B6, which aids your nervous and immune systems.

The potato's fiber, potassium, vitamin C, and vitamin B6 content, coupled with its lack of cholesterol, all support heart health. Potatoes contain significant amounts of fiber. Fiber helps lower the total amount of cholesterol in the blood, thereby decreasing the risk of heart disease.

SARDINES

Sardines contain 20 grams of protein per three-ounce serving, and are one of the best sources of calcium and vitamin D, both of which are essential for bone and muscle health. They're high in omega-3 fatty acids, which help fight inflammation and lower LDL (bad) cholesterol. They might have workout benefits to boot.

Sardines contain 20 grams of protein per three-ounce serving, and are one of the best sources of calcium and vitamin D, both of which are essential for bone and muscle health.

They're high in omega-3 fatty acids, which help fight inflammation and lower LDL (bad) cholesterol. They might have workout benefits to boot. Researchers from Saint Louis University found that athletes who took an omega-3 supplement before and after arm curls felt less sore than those who'd had a placebo.

BLUEBERRIES

All berries are good for your health. They're loaded with antioxidants, which help your arteries relax and may have anti-aging effects as well. But for men especially, blueberries are king. Blueberries have lots of vitamin K, which helps your blood clot, and plenty of vitamin C like most berries.

A daily bowl could protect against obesity, heart disease and diabetes. A bowl of wild blueberries a day could protect against a range of health problems including obesity, heart disease and diabetes. Berries are rich in polyphenols – antioxidants that protect cells in the heart and help lower blood pressure.

AVOCADOS

Avocado is rich in folic acid for increased energy production, along with healthy fats to improve mood and sense of well-being. The more avocado you consume, the more blood flow your body experiences — which is useful when it comes to sexual performance and in turn will also help lower the risk of heart disease.

Avocados are a great source of vitamins C, E, K, and B-6, as well as riboflavin, niacin, folate, pantothenic acid, magnesium, and potassium. They also provide lutein, beta-carotene, and omega-3 fatty acids. Although most of the calories in an avocado come from fat, don't shy away!

WHOLE GRAINS

Foods such as wheat, rice, oats, cornmeal, barley, quinoa or products made from these foods are considered grains. Grains are high in carbohydrates which provide energy to your brain and muscles. Not all grains are created equally in terms of nutritional benefits. The health benefits of a grain depend on the form of the grain you actually eat. There are two types of grains: whole grains and refined grains.

When you eat a whole grain, your body is getting nutrients found in all parts of the grain, as well as fiber. Whole grain foods include oatmeal, brown rice, quinoa, and whole wheat bread or pasta. Refined grains have been processed and are missing some nutrients. Refined grain foods include white bread, white rice, and many kinds of pasta. When you eat grains, try having whole grains as much as possible.

A GLASS OF RED WINE

A study from 2019 reports that males who drank alcohol had a slightly lower risk of lethal prostate cancer, and that red wine had links with a lower risk of progression to lethal disease. The authors say that these results mean moderate alcohol consumption is safe for people with prostate cancer.

The health benefits from wine are the same for men and women, but men can drink more given their generally larger body mass — one or two 4-ounce glasses of wine per day — while women should consume only one glass.

WATERMELON

Watermelon may be a natural Viagra, says a researcher. That's because the popular summer fruit is richer than experts believed in an amino acid called citrulline, which relaxes and dilates blood vessels much like Viagra and other drugs meant to treat erectile dysfunction (ED).

Watermelon is a natural source of citrulline. Citrulline is an amino acid that may support better erections. Viagra works by increasing blood flow to the penis, allowing a man to more easily get an erection when he is aroused. Citrulline may do the same thing, although it works in a different way to Viagra.

Chapter Four

How To Build Blood for Good Erection

In this chapter, I will expose you to four ingredient that are needed to build blood in the body system needed for good erection.

Chlorophyll:

So, with the information that red platelets are produced in the small bowel and that they are formed from the food we eat, it will be clear that the nature of the food we eat will dramatically affect the nature of the red blood cells being produced. Regardless of whether the small intestine is absolutely healthy to such an extent that the blood-creating organs is unblemished, it is still truly essential to eat food sources which contain heathy ingredients.

Chlophyll is plant blood. For commonsense purposes chlorophyll is the substance which causes plants to seem green. It has a similar structure as haemoglobin which is the piece of our platelets liable for holding oxygen. A researcher and they ought to be exceptionally amazed and can't help thinking about why they were rarely aware about the insignificant difference between chlorophyll and haemoglobin. This implies that our blood structure is the same with that of leaves and grass. We were not told this in school. The only tangible difference between chlorophyl and haemoglobin is that the nucleus part of haemoglobin is iron but that of chlorophyll is magnesium. The body can without much effort convert the blood of plants, into human blood, thus eating/drinking greens is like transfusion of blood, which means higher volume, better quality and more oxygen-rich platelets. Better blood means more energy, better wellbeing and healthy erection. Chlorophyll will likewise invigorate and resuscitate existing cells.

Basically, healthy erection is sure, if you can increase blood volume by taking a tablespoon of fluid chlorophyll like World Organic, Dsouza's, or the pH Miracle brand, in 4 oz. of ionized water, all day long. On the off chance that you don't eat/drink greens the body should make do and 'Improvise' new cells out of whatever materials are accessible.

Green food sources are the way to progress for such countless reasons and the more significant the amount of greens you devour, the more noteworthy the medical advantages you get. Grown grasses and their juices are a great wellspring of concentrated chlorophyll. Green in general, particularly grasses are alkalizing, high in amino acids and anti-fungal (the protein you get wheat grass is four times more than that of meat). An additional advantage of these food sources is the bounty of nutrients and alkaline minerals important to support acids, recuperate the small digestive system and feed the whole body. Greens likewise cleanse the liver and blood and chlorophyll will assist with securing you against substantial metals, electrical contamination and oxidative pressure.

People can eat grass, however it should be mixed, squeezed or dried and transformed into powder. Human teeth are a significant successful 'wheatgrass juicer', you can simply bite a chunk of grass for some time, then dispose the mash when there is no flavour left. This implies freshly squeezed in your mouth with no opportunity for it to oxidize as it does when put through a mechanical juicer. Wheatgrass Juice which contains chlorophyll, nutrients, minerals and supplements has been connected to numerous health advantages, which also include building blood for erection.

Oil or Lipids or Good fats

Another ingredient for building blood for erection is an healthy, essential oil. While chlorophyll create oxygen carrying part of the red blood cells, raw and uncooked essential oil or fat create a strong and flexible membrane for the red blood cells.

If you consume a lot of fats and green, you can maintain a good circulatory system.

Water:

Does this look casual? Yes, it may. Oh, like the normal motivation to drink at least 4 litres of water in a day. This ingredient is very important to maintain good erection. It refreshes and cleanse the blood stream for healthy and hydrated new cells. For high energy level blood, you need water.

Salt:

The body uses salt to produce sodium bicarbonate, iron and other minerals. This helps a great deal to neutralize acid and maintain healthy PH balance. Salt is also important in our body system in blood circulation processes. Unprocessed salt is very good than table salt.

Chapter Five

DOES VIAGRA HELPS?

VIAGRA, as a brand name of **sildenafil citrate,** is an erectile dysfunction drug and can also be called phosphodiesterase type 5 (PDE 5) inhibitors. It performs its function by relaxing the blood vessels in the manhood (*your penis*), allowing free and unobstructed movement of blood to the penis when you get excited sexually.

It was produced by a group of pharmaceutical chemists working at Pfizer's Sandwich. The research of this drug was initially for the treatment of high blood pressure (hypertension) and the occurrence of ischaemic heart disease called angina pectoris. The result of this study led to a suggestion by Ian Osterloh, that the pill will have a little effect on a patient with angina pectoris, but will trigger the effect of penile erection. This suggestion led to the redirection of their initial intention and made Pfizer decided to sell the drug for erectile dysfunction, rather than for angina.

The drug was authorized for production in 1996 and was approved for use on the treatment of erectile dysfunction by the FDA in March 1998, becoming the first oral treatment approved in the united states to treat erectile dysfunction, and offered for sale in that same year. Gradually the purchase of Viagra increases annually and maintain a great success in 2008 as it reaches an annual deal of US$1.934 billion.

Peter Dunn and Albert Wood were recorded as the inventors of the drug, but for the original composition of matter patent Andrew Bell, David Brown, and Nicholas Terrett are listed.

Viagra has played an essential role as a revolutionary drug for erectile dysfunction. It helps men everywhere who are suffering from erectile dysfunction to be able to maintain an erection. Erectile dysfunction poses a grave problem for two sexual partners, and it is common among elderly sexual partners. As a man increases in age, the chances of having erectile dysfunction also increase. Over time, men having this issue struggles all through during sexual activities to gain erection, in which they have always been disappointed.

Now, regarding this sickness, Viagra is one of the solution drugs which has been provided to help men suffering from ED to gain erection actively.

The use of Viagra

VIAGRA is used for the treatment of erectile dysfunction (also known to be Impotence). This is a situation when a man cannot get or maintain a firm or hard, erection suitable enough for sexual activity.

The compositional Ingredients of Viagra?

The following are the composition element of Viagra;

- *Sildenafil citrate:* This is the primary or active component of Viagra. Base on categories, each tablet contains 25mg, 50mg,100mg of sildenafil citrate. The primary active ingredient in Viagra is *Sildenafil citrate*, which is the secret of how and why this drug works effectively. Sildenafil citrate is a white to off-white crystalline powder with a solubility profile dependent on ph. In its solid-state, it is considered to be extremely stable, as demonstrated by data derived from forced degradation studies. It is stable at 90°C in an inert atmosphere. This is to indicate the significant compound use during the composition or production of Viagra.

- **Tablet core:** it is composed of Calcium hydrogen phosphate, Microcrystalline cellulose, Magnesium stearate, Croscarmellose sodium.
- **Film Coat:** it is composed of Hypromellose, Titanium dioxide(E171), Aluminium Lake (E132), Triacetin, indigo carmine.

How long does it take to start the effect?

Generally, based on the composition of Viagra, it should begin its effect thirty (30) minutes after use. But this effect varies from individual to individual because of body chemistry, but irrespective of the body composition, it must begin to work at most sixty (60) minutes.

How long does Viagra take to maintain effect?

The time it takes after use also varies from individual to individual. But the effect starts to reduce from 2-3 hours after it begins work when taken. Although it was composed to work for 5 hours at length when used with some sexual stimulants.

Some specific factors may affect the period Viagra is to last after its effect starts in an individual, but this will be discussed below. It is highly advisable to know and consult your doctor before use or start a course of remedy with Viagra.

Factors that may affect the lasting effect of Viagra and some other ED drugs

The following are some factors that may add up or reduce the period that it will take Viagra and some other ED drugs to be active when they are used. Some of these factors are discussed below. Paraventure, your expectations towards the long-lasting effect of Viagra were cut short; check out these factors in you before given your review or conclusion on the impact of the drug.

- *Age*

The more a man grows older (increases in years), the more the body metabolism slows down. This implies that Men over 65 years of age will find Viagra stays in their body system for a long time because of the slow metabolism of their body system. Hence, the older you grow, the more the effect of Viagra lasts longer in your body, or better still Viagra last long in impact on older people.

- *Alcohol*

Consumption of alcohol decreases the flow of blood to the penis; this causes the penis to find it hard to gain an erection. Thereby reduces the effect of Viagra on the penis.

- *Diet*

Food with a high content of fat takes the body more time and hard work to digest. Now, the consumption of this type of food will only take Viagra a long time to begin effect or start working, because the body system will be busy digesting the food. But taking these pills without food in the stomach will make the start effect quickly.

- *Dosage*

As per the categories of Viagra tablet, we have Viagra 25mg, 50mg, 100mg of sildenafil citrate. The higher the type you get as to the quantity of sildenafil citrate, the more effective and long-lasting the effect will be. Consult your doctor for the right prescription of the dosage suitable for you. But the appropriate dosage is 50mg.

- *Drug interactions*

Specific medication can affect the effectiveness of Viagra, such as the use of antibiotic rifampicin for the treatment of tuberculosis. The proper thing to take note is to discuss with your doctor any medicine you are using at that particular time to be able to know, and maybe it is wise to take Viagra or not.

- *Smoking*

Men who smoke cigarettes are also liable to sexual imbalances. Smoking is one of the possible causes of erectile dysfunction because it destroys blood vessels, and erectile dysfunction is caused by an inadequate flow of blood to the penile organ. Someone who smokes is forty per cent likely to have erectile dysfunction when compared to one who doesn't smoke.

- *Health condition*.

The condition of your health depends on how properly this drug will function or be useful in your body system. It is advisable to visit your doctor for a proper check-up before use.

- *Timing of Administration*

Viagra should typically be taken about 30 minutes to 1 hour before sexual activity. Taking it too long before or after a meal can affect its absorption and onset of action. Following the instructions provided by your healthcare professional or the medication label is important for optimal results.

Precaution on the right dose of Viagra

For most erectile dysfunction patients, the recommended dose of **VIAGRA** is 50 mg taken as needed. If necessary, to increase or decrease the treatment, your doctor will be the best person to listen to because he/ she understands the chemistry of your body system. The maximum dose you can take is 100 mg, and the minimum 25 mg if required.

Follow your doctor's instructions on the use of *Viagra*. Take this pill 30 – 60 minutes before the start of the sexual activity. If you are confused about the right dosage, notify your doctor. Take medicine by swallowing it, pushing it down with water. Do not chew the pill for effectiveness.

Note: if peradventure you take Viagra before sex, DO NOT USE VIAGRA MORE THAN ONCE A DAY.

Irrespective of the type you are taking, be it 25mg or 50mg or 100mg. It is required that you use ONE (1) pill per day. If more is required, your doctor or the pharmacist will let you know.

Precautions on when Not to Take Viagra or any other ED Drugs

The following are the warnings you are advised to heed to before you take or take a step of buying Viagra or any other ED drugs. Most of the precautions are the same for other ED drugs.

- You must not take Viagra when you are on Nitrates or Nitrite medications. This may lead to an excessive drop in your blood pressure, and you may not find it easy for treatment. This is because sexual activity places a lot of strain on the heart.

- Refrain from Viagra if you are been treated for chest pain (angina) or some other heart condition that get you using medications called nitrate.

- Refrain from Viagra if you are using *guanylate cyclase stimulator (GCS),* for example, *Adepmas* known as *riociguat.* GCS is a type of medicine that is used for the treatment of *chronic thromboembolic pulmonary hypertension (CTEPH)* or *pulmonary arterial hypertension (PAH)*. *CTEPH* is high blood pressure in the blood vessels in the lungs caused by blood clots in the lungs, while *PAH* is narrowing of the vessels that carry blood from the heart to the lungs.

- Do not take Viagra if you have been diagnosed with a stroke or heart attack for like six (6) months.

- Patients with liver problems should abstain from Viagra.

- When a patient is having eye diseases, such as retinitis pigmentosa, and non-arteritis anterior ischaemic optic neuropathy (NAION).

- Do not take Viagra when the packaging is turned, or you noticed a sign of opening.

- Check the expiry date, maybe be it hasn't passed the manufacturer period assigned for it for use. If it has, please kindly return it to the pharmacist or throw it away.

Health conditions that may prevent you from using Viagra.

The following are the health issues that prevent a man from using Viagra.

- A disease of the blood called sickle cell anemia

- Kidney or liver problems

- Diabetes, especially if you also have eye problems

- Color vision problems

- Any bleeding disorder such as hemophilia

- Previously experienced a sudden decrease or loss of hearing.

- Leukemia (cancer of the blood cells)

- Multiple myelomas (a cancer of the bone marrow)

- Any disease or deformity of your penis

- Stomach ulcer

Drugs that Interact with Viagra?

The following medicines can interact with the use of Viagra.

- Some antibiotics like erythromycin and rifampicin

- Drugs called alpha-blockers; these are used for the treatment of high blood pressure or prostate problems.

- Tracleer (bosentan), a medicine used to treat high blood pressure in the vessels of the lungs.

- Cimetidine, a medicine used to treat ulcers

- Some medicines used to treat fungal infections including ketoconazole and itraconazole

- Some protease inhibitors such as ritonavir and saquinavir for the treatment of HIV infection

What to do when you take an overdose?

Immediate you discover that you have taken an overdose, rush to see your doctor or call poison information centre

(PIC). It takes less than 20 minutes before the severe reaction starts. Even though the effect has not started, take a drastic measure to either seeing your doctor or call PIC.

Is Viagra safe for health?

Viagra is safe for use, when you are healthy, when you are not on medications that can alter some adverse reaction in the body, and your body system is not suffering from the earlier mentioned diseases.

What Are the Possible Side Effects of Viagra?

Side effect or adverse reactions are some experiences have gotten, contrary to the significant expectations or functions of a particular drug.

As we all know to other drugs or medicines, side effects can not be sidelined, VIAGRA also causes side effects, although not everybody gets them. The side effects obtained from Viagra are usually controlled and doesn't take a long time. All medicine without the exception of Viagra can cause allergic reactions. Base on this, it is wise if you contact your doctor immediately. Do not take self medications like, for example, and If peradventure you have chest pains during or after intercourse, relaxation is the best solution to that, do not think of taking Nitrates to treat the effect, it may eventually lead to what you cannot handle. Reach your doctor as soon as possible.

The following symptoms should be acted upon for complaints if you discovered after the use of Viagra:

- Sudden wheeziness,

- Difficulty in breathing.

- Dizziness

- Swelling of the eyelids, face, lips, or throat.

- When you have a long time and sometimes painful erections, this has been reported after taking VIAGRA.

If you noticed your erection lasts for more than 4 hours after the use of Viagra, see a doctor immediately.

- A sudden decrease or loss of vision.

You must see your doctor if you noticed any of these symptoms after the use of Viagra.

The most common side effect of Viagra

Ranging from 1 – 10 patients, the most common side effect that more than one person will complain about after the use of Viagra is a headache.

The common side effect of Viagra

These are some common side effects that may likely happen after the use of Viagra.

- Headache: This is one of the most frequently reported side effects of Viagra. It can range from mild to moderate in intensity.

- Flushing: Some individuals may experience facial flushing or redness, often accompanied by a feeling of warmth. This is caused by increased blood flow to the face.

- Indigestion and Upset Stomach: Viagra can cause gastrointestinal symptoms such as indigestion, stomach discomfort, and acid reflux.

- Nasal Congestion: Some people may experience a stuffy or runny nose after taking Viagra.

- Dizziness: Viagra can occasionally cause dizziness or light-headedness, particularly when standing up quickly. It's important to avoid activities that require mental alertness if you experience this side effect.

- Visual Disturbances: Rarely, Viagra may cause mild and temporary changes in vision, such as a blue tinge to vision or increased sensitivity to light.

- Back Pain and Muscle Aches: Some individuals may experience muscle aches, including back pain, after taking Viagra. These side effects are usually mild and resolve on their own.

It's important to note that these side effects are generally mild and temporary. However, if any of these side effects persist or worsen, it's advisable to seek medical attention. Additionally, there are rare but serious side effects associated with Viagra, such as priapism (prolonged erection), sudden vision loss, and allergic reactions.

Uncommon side effect

There has been some record of some side effects which are not common but happens. These may be likely to occur out of 1000 patients, like 1-10. The following are the list of some of these effects, in case if it probably happens.

- Dry mouth.

- Chest pain.

- Feeling tired.

- Muscle pain.

- Nausea.

- Vomiting.

- Skin rash.

- Bleeding at the back of the eye.

- Bloodshot eyes/red eyes.

- Vertigo Abnormal sensation in the eye.

- Irregular or rapid heartbeat.

- Vertigo.

- Feeling sleepy.

- Reduced sense of touch.

- Vertigo

- Ringing in the ears.

Rare side effects

These occur once in every ten thousand, i.e., it is scarce

before you hear of this kind of side effect.

- High blood pressure.

- Low blood pressure.

- Fainting.

- Stroke.

- Nosebleed.

- Sudden decrease.

- Loss of hearing.

- Pounding heartbeat.

- Chest pain.

- Sudden death.

- Heart attack or temporary decreased blood flow to parts of the brain.

Which is safer

Summarily, the figure below shows some effect of Viagra on the body system.

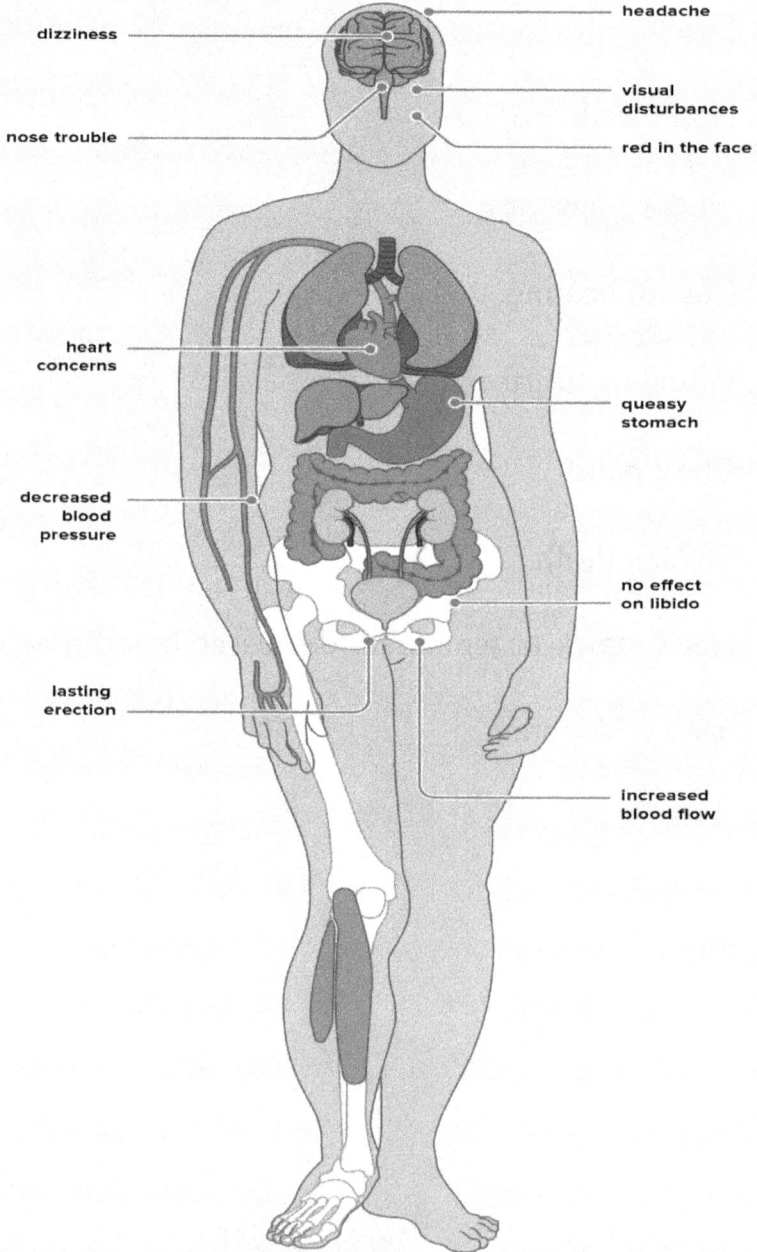

About the *Author*

Fred Wright is a Writer, Publisher, and medical practitioner. Over the past three decades, he has worked in a wide variety of professional capacities in both the private and public sectors. He has been able to help a lot of people treat different health issues ranging from internal to external diseases.

Acknowledgements

First of all, my appreciation goes to God Almighty for the opportunity to collate this manuscript. And lastly, to all who supported me in kinds and cash, in ideas and design. May God bless you all.

www.ingramcontent.com/pod-product-compliance
Lightning Source LLC
Chambersburg PA
CBHW060255030426
42335CB00014B/1706